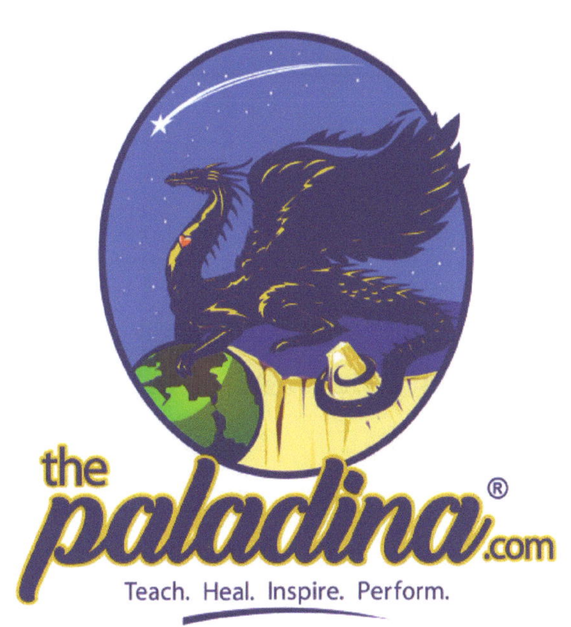
the
paladina®
.com
Teach. Heal. Inspire. Perform.

Bad Shot? ASAP: Detox! Large Print

2024 © Christine Padovan
2024 © Paladina International
Published by Paladina International
ISBN 9798326603159
Copyright data is available on file.
Padovan, Christine, 1961-

    I. Health & Wellness   II. Title

https://thepaladina.com
https://heavymetalpoisoning.org

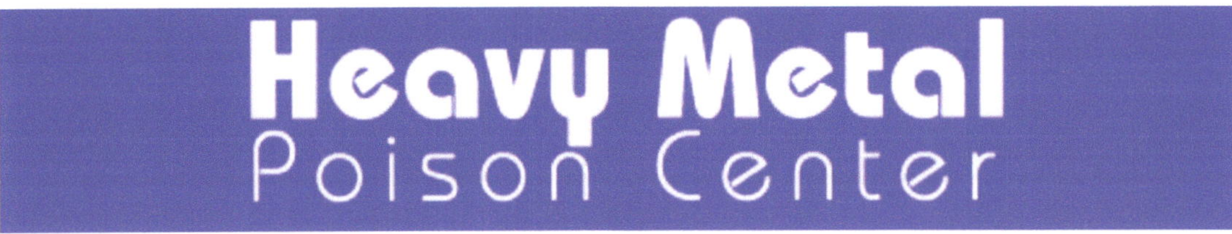

Bad Shot? ASAP: Detox! Large Print is compiled according to the best practices and guidelines for Large Print Documents used by the Low Vision Community authored by the Council of Citizens with Low Vision International An Affiliate of the American Council of the Blind, Arlington, VA. www.cclvi.org

Cover art by·Vicki White.

Bad Shot?

ASAP: Detox! Large Print

How My Own Poisoning Revealed the Truth About the Covid Shots

by Christine Padovan

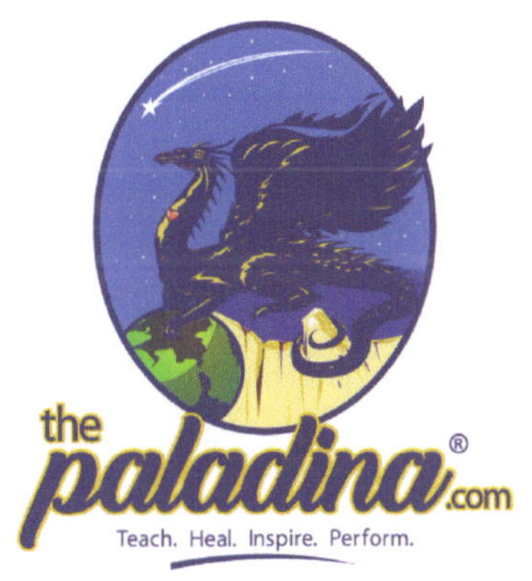

Paladina International
Orlando, Florida USA
in the year 2024

Dedication:

For humanity and all living

beings on Earth

Table of Contents

Acknowledgements

One doesn't write a book, a booklet, an article or a paragraph without getting some sort of inspiration, encouragement, learning or assistance from somewhere or someone.

Thank you to Dr. Hildegarde Staninger, RIET-1 Industrial Toxicologist/ IH & Doctor of Integrative Medicine for saving my life and the lives of countless others with your knowledge on toxins, chemicals and poisons, on nano technology and current military and commercial experiments, in teaching natural and safe detoxification, and your ability to analysis forensic toxicity tests that most other university-trained toxicology professors and practitioners cannot seem to do.

The field of toxicology is sorely lacking in brilliant minds like Dr. Staninger. I hope we can start putting together the needed coursework to get up and coming toxicology majors and future toxicologists up to speed on chronic toxicity build-up versus acute poisoning, and how heavy metals and chemicals do not just 'go away' on their own once inside the body without help. Also, the role of nano technology and how it can be used for good, but more often than not, is abused as we have seen with recent criminal poisoning cases and what is going on with vaccine injections.

Thank you to Mr. Kaily Bissani and Dr. Zack Bissani of The Carlson Company Labs for your informative website https://thecarlsoncompany. net/ and for educating me on Gas Chromatography and Mass Spectrometry, and how using both forensic methods in all testing, makes sure any nano technology is bypassed and all elements are fully revealed.

I'd also like to thank my father, the late Antonio Padovan for making me the intuitive, smartass I am today, and my mother Agnes Padovan for being the kind, gentle soul she is and showing how the world can be a better place by just being sweet and loving to everyone you meet.

To my gifted colleague, Michael Lombard who received confirmation spiritually as I did several days ago that I needed to get out this vital information to the masses sooner rather than later (my new national radio show hasn't started yet, and a Rumble.com channel and a podcast can only reach so many people at a time).

And to my friends, M & B Brooks and in 2023, M & L Davis, my gratitude in providing a temporary place to live while between homes is greater than you can ever know.

> • • • <

Introduction

Many of you have seen what is happening in the world. Since around December 2019, news started to leak out of China that a new coronavirus called SARS-CoV-2 (SARS stands for Severe Acute Respiratory Syndrome) was rapidly making its way through the town of Wuhan. This new coronavirus, afterwards dubbed 'Covid-19' was reported to be making the rounds in China at a rapid rate, and then the first case appeared in Washington State in January 2020.

At the time, that was the least of my concerns. I had been poisoned badly with large doses of heavy metals for the fourth and final time (twice had been indirectly through sex with my ex loved one – also a poisoned victim - and twice directly by the suspects) in October 2019.

Large amounts of arsenic were snuck into my coffee mug by my ex-lover between October 22 and 25, and then I later discovered while both of us had been off the property on October 19th, our trailer's water tank which was not locked at the time had been tainted with heavy metals.

The goal was to get my ex-lover to bump me off by slow poisoning him through an ex-girlfriend they put in front of him in the summer of 2018 – the thallium and other metals made it easy to manipulate his thinking, an already very naïve, distrusting person to begin with, and convince him I was the problem, not them or his ex.

The suspects who I knew well and had even figured out with intuitive abilities, behavior observations, conversations, texts/emails and science tested evidence between 2013 and 2018 who their associates were and the family members they brainwashed into joining them, had tried very hard one final time in bumping me off. Why? I had several criminal cases open on them and on one of their associates and a family member with police, and evidence, forensic tests, tips and information shared with the FBI through police and myself.

So I had to recover by detoxifying yet again to reverse the food allergies, the kidney and heart damage, the out-of-control intestinal tract, the nerve damage without going to the hospital, even though this time, I was in way more serious shape.

Why not go to the hospital? Because I already knew from our forensic tests I had paid for out of pocket in 2017 and 2018 (Anthem Blue Cross of CA does not cover anything toxicology) and a loved one's hospital tests that regular hospital tests would not show any poisoning because nano technology was being used to keep barely anything from being seen on a regular doctor or hospital test.

And I didn't have the forensic results yet for my then current October 2019 poisoning which would take up to 10 days to get from the lab I was then using. I also knew our suspects formerly and currently worked in the medical and pharmaceutical fields, and that if I went into the hospital, they would make sure I would not come out alive. Even Dr. Staninger, in the know by her involvement as an expert witness on poisoning cases said 'whatever you do, don't go to the hospital!' She didn't have to tell me but she did anyway.

Game over if I had gone in – no one else would make sure to eventually stop these people if I died – and they very well knew that.

> • • • <

Bad Shot? ASAP: Detox!   p 10

Chapter 1:
The Connection to Covid-19 and the 'vaccines'

So you are now going to ask 'OK, Christine. What does any of this have to do with Covid-19?' Great question. As I was slowly and painfully recovering from that major poisoning (see my November 2019 forensic test below – since the poisoning was recent, I sent in my urine for testing), Dr. Staninger and I were always in touch periodically, and one conversation had to do with the Covid-19 'vaccine' shots when they were about to become available.

First, I'll describe what I was going through to recover and remove the heavy metals as quickly as possible from my body without doing further damage or harm to me.

It took me at least 8 weeks for my body to start having its own control of my bowel movements. I literally had NO CONTROL of my bowel movements. Meaning if I felt a fart coming on, it would not just be a fart. It would have something 'additional' to it and I couldn't just keep soiling my underwear. I had to do something to assist me in slowing and controlling the diarrhea while I was starting a new job as a field investigator (yes, I literally was working full -time while detoxifying – very difficult to do but I had to do it).

For sure, I knew any gastro-intestinal doctor was going to prescribe Prednisone as a now former loved one had been prescribed and I saw how bad his body had become reliant on it because he had refused to be diligent with detoxifying when I begged him to. Prednisone is a steroid and you do not want to stay on it long term. I opted to take a full adult dose of Pepto Bismol in the morning when I got up, and a full adult dose of it at night. That assisted me in keeping the diarrhea under control, though I still had to be near a toilet for at least the first month because when I felt I had to go, I had to go!

I was taking 4000mg a day of reduced glutathione – 2000mg in the morning and 2000 mg in the evening daily for the first 3 weeks (I used the Nusapure brand off Amazon; also our family had done detoxing using other brands, including the aSquared brand – capsules are smaller and easier for older folks to swallow. Nusapure and aSquared are quality and very affordable). Now, you'll say – 'Christine, isn't that a large amount to take?'

In a sense, yes – but glutathione is water soluble like Vitamin C. You can easily take up to 10 grams of Vitamin C a day when you have a cold you want to get rid of and you are fine. Though anything past 10 grams in 24 hours can make you a little 'loose' downstairs. So, I was not worried at all.

Glutathione is in every cell of our body, and I needed strong protection from the amount of toxicity I had in my body to protect my heart and brain. It is neutralizing the acidity of the body, putting a protective coating around the toxins, in my case – metals – and gently pulling them out of the body.

I also took 1200mg of fish oil (Omega 3's) daily with my other vitamins for added brain protection and 600 mg of activated charcoal before bed for added detoxification assistance. I also made Dr. Staninger's recipe for Bay Leaf Water and drank lots of that daily for a liquid version of glutathione to rinse my organs, especially the kidneys and liver.

THE CARLSON COMPANY INC
Call: 1-866-889-3410 or email: carlsonco@comcast.net

Client: **Carlson Company LLC** Addr: **10343 Federal Blvd Ste J-401** **Westminster, CO 80260** Phone: **(719) 531-6666** Contact: **Kaily Bissani**	First Name: **Christine** Last Name: **Padovan** ID: **N/A** Test Name: **Comprehensive Metal Test** Profile: **UCC2049** Media: **Urine** Reason: **Other**	Specid: **Christine** Acc #: **193040007** Collected: **10/25/2019** Received: **10/31/2019 10:19 AM** Released: **11/25/2019 2:13 PM** Status: **Complete**

Substance	Lab Result	Test Value		High Value	Test Method
LITHIUM	Detected	61 ug/L		200 ug/L	ICPMS
BERYLLIUM	Detected	0.072 ug/L		2 ug/L	ICPMS
ALUMINUM	Detected	17 ug/L		30 ug/L	ICPMS
CHROMIUM	Detected	1.9 ug/L		40 ug/L	ICPMS
MANGANESE	Detected	1.2 ug/L	H	1 ug/L	ICPMS
COBALT	Detected	2.1 ug/L	H	2 ug/L	ICPMS
NICKEL	Detected	3.0 ug/L		4 ug/L	ICPMS
COPPER	Detected	9.7 ug/L		75 ug/L	ICPMS
ZINC	Detected	551 ug/L		1300 ug/L	ICPMS
ARSENIC	Detected	604 ug/L	H	35 ug/L	ICPMS
SELENIUM	Detected	25 ug/L		200 ug/L	ICPMS
SILVER	< 0.01 ug/L	< 0.01 ug/L		100 ug/L	ICPMS
CADMIUM	Detected	0.21 ug/L		3 ug/L	ICPMS
TIN	Detected	0.59 ug/L		17 ug/L	ICPMS
ANTIMONY	Detected	0.29 ug/L		3.6 ug/L	ICPMS
BARIUM	Detected	5.3 ug/L		20 ug/L	ICPMS
PLATINUM	Detected	0.030 ug/L		0.03 ug/L	ICPMS
MERCURY	Detected	10 ug/L		20 ug/L	ICPMS
LEAD	Detected	0.12 ug/L		80 ug/L	ICPMS
THORIUM	Detected	0.11 ug/L		3.8 ug/L	ICPMS
URANIUM	< 0.01 ug/L	< 0.01 ug/L		0.3 ug/L	ICPMS
TITANIUM	Detected	249 µg/L	H	1 µg/L	ICPMS
VANADIUM	Detected	0.89 µg/L	H	0.2 µg/L	ICPMS
RUBIDIUM	Detected	756 µg/L	H	0.01 µg/L	ICPMS
MOLYBDENUM	Detected	94 µg/L	H	2.0 µg/L	ICPMS
STRONTIUM	Detected	541 µg/L	H	144 µg/L	ICPMS
GADOLINIUM	< 0.01 µg/L	< 0.01 µg/L		0.2 µg/L	ICPMS
THALLIUM	Detected	1.4 µg/L	H	0.4 µg/L	ICPMS
BISMUTH	Detected	17 µg/L	H	0.5 µg/L	ICPMS
TUNGSTEN	Detected	0.35 µg/L	H	0.08 µg/L	ICPMS

Test Comment:

The preceding result has been reviewed and is certified to be as reported. <u>Brandon Cox</u> (Certifying Scientist)

End of Report	Laboratory Director: Ernest D. Lykissa, Ph.D. Forensic Toxicologist Print Date: 11/25/2019 16:48:06	Page 1 of 1

After 3 weeks, I reduced the amount of glutathione to 2000mg a day. 1000mg in the morning and 1000mg in the evening. I was able to start slowing down on the amount of Pepto Bismol I took after week 4.

My advice is to be guided by your body as it starts to regain control of its bowel movements. Also, be aware that the cramping of muscles, as well as thumb muscles, calf muscles and internal muscles you never thought could cramp will be excruciating and you will need a bottle of Potassium (99mg tablets or capsules) handy to take as soon as you feel one coming on.

My body is naturally low in potassium (my inherited blood on my father's side – low potassium and low iron), so as a lifelong athlete, I always have a bottle of potassium in my vitamin cabinet and have been taking one (1) 99 mg tablet daily my whole adult life to keep calf and feet/toe cramps away. But when detoxifying from the high doses of arsenic, thallium and the 13 other metals in high quantities in my body, the cramping could literally happen out of nowhere and was extremely painful and sometimes, temporarily debilitating.

Why does this happen? Unfortunately, an element such as thallium (which by the way, has been illegal in the USA since 1980) has a similar molecular structure to potassium, so the body is fooled into thinking the thallium is potassium and easily says 'hey, come on in!' Then your body starts to rebel when the thallium does its dirty work. Thus, your body now is needing real, extra potassium to combat the cramping.

However, you know "this too shall pass" so you have to unfortunately weather through all of this as you are detoxifying, reversing temporary allergies (I could not eat any wheat, gluten, dairy and most nuts during this time) and healing my organs, my brain, my heart, my mind and body back to optimal health.

Additional supportive detoxifying was done with Infrared sauna therapy and hyperbaric oxygen sessions. Also, meditation and positive thinking in knowing I would fully recover were key factors as well.

After a full 8 weeks had past, which was by Christmas time 2019, my bowels were back in control again and Pepto Bismol was used sparingly. To continue gentle detoxification, I then went to 500mg twice a day of glutathione for another 3 months, then back down to the standard daily adult dose of 500mg a day.

Ok, you go – 'that explains what you were doing to get the toxins out of you. What has this to do with Covid-19 and the shots?'

Absolutely, everything.

> • • • <

Bad Shot? ASAP: Detox! p 16

Chapter 2:
The connection to Covid-19, the shots and Glutathione

As I was detoxifying, Covid-19 cases were ramping up in the United States and basically, all over the world. I was still in California at the time and in March 2020, Governor Newsom became the first governor to impose lockdown measurements.

Personally, this didn't affect me because as of mid-February 2020, I was back to working as a Flex security guard for what is now Allied Universal. I had to work full-time outside of my career as a voice artist to keep paying off credit card bills that accumulated after years of paying for toxicology analysis and consults, forensic testing and detoxification treatments. Security guards were exempt from lockdown because guards were needed to keep buildings secure, especially when no employees were there.

However, there were precautions we had to take. Wearing a surgical mask became mandatory on job sites, even if no employees were around. We had to wear nitrile gloves when checking inside or outside doors to make sure they were secure and we weren't leaving our germs on the door handles. Then as you know, supermarkets and other establishments made it mandatory for anyone entering to wear a face mask. I don't have to tell you more – you all know the story.

Was I concerned about catching Covid-19? Actually, no. Here's why. I knew from reading about glutathione since I had been on it since 2017, that not only was it a master detoxifier, it was also an immunity booster. It had first been studied in 1970 by an Italian doctor (sorry, still cannot find the original study yet) who wanted to know a natural way to boost the immune system of the elderly against pneumonia. He found that boosting the levels of glutathione in the body, which naturally decrease in production as we get older, kept the elderly from succumbing to pneumonia. So I took it daily and still do.

Imagine this. Here it was 2020 and a natural element, in medical use in IVs and suppositories and as a food grade supplement was known since 1970 as a viral protector besides being a master detoxifier! The first studies actually came out in May 2020, touting the science that indeed, low glutathione levels in the body were the most likely reason for how severe the Covid-19 case would be for that person and also most likely lead to death:

Endogenous Deficiency of Glutathione as the Most Likely Cause of Serious Manifestations and Death in COVID-19 Patients

- Alexey Polonikov*

Cite this: *ACS Infect. Dis.* 2020, 6, 7, 1558–1562
Publication Date: May 28, 2020
https://doi.org/10.1021/acsinfecdis.0c00288
Copyright © 2020 American Chemical Society

Link to study:
https://pubs.acs.org/doi/10.1021/acsinfecdis.0c00288
Another study came out in July 2020, again showing that effective levels of glutathione protect and assist in recovery from Covid-19:
Antioxidants (Basel). 2020 Jul; 9(7): 624.
Published online 2020 Jul 16. doi: 10.3390/antiox9070624
PMCID: PMC7402141
PMID: 32708578

The Role of Glutathione in Protecting against the Severe Inflammatory Response Triggered by COVID-19

Francesca Silvagno,[*] Annamaria Vernone, and Gian Piero Pescarmona

Link to study:
https://www.ncbi.nlm.nih.gov/pmc/articles/PMC7402141/
(More studies and websites have since come out, touting glutathione.)

Dr. Richard Horowitz, a Lyme disease specialist, quietly was saving and protecting his Covid-19 patients when he discovered the key was adding glutathione to his treatment protocol. He lists his protocols on a special page on his website and his severe Covid treatment actually makes a great detox treatment as well (by the way, only one local news station ever interviewed him about it):

https://www.lymedisease.org/pfeiffer-preventing-covid/

Because I proved my mother was full of heavy metal toxins (one main suspect in particular was targeting my mother at her assisted living place in NJ, primarily through one nurses aide), I had my mother since February 2019 on glutathione to gently detoxify her, as I continued to work to make my way eventually out of California and away from my then loved one's family connections to these suspects and quietly work the cases. I couldn't afford to spend thousands of dollars on a Carlson Company lab test for my mom (credit cards were basically full), so I used a Doctors Data hair full panel heavy metal toxicity test kit from Directlabs.com through Dr. Staninger's connection with them.

These Doctors Data heavy metal and chemical toxicity forensic tests range from 112.00 to 169.00, depending on the discount you get through a particular referral or online coupon and if you test for hair or urine; metals or chemicals. The Doctors Data tests use the same forensic modality in their tests to test for heavy metals as do other forensic labs (which is "inductively coupled plasma mass spectrometry (ICP-MS), a type of mass spectrometry that uses an inductively coupled plasma to ionize the sample. It atomizes the sample and creates atomic and small polyatomic ions, which are then detected." (Wikipedia).

A slight problem – Direct Labs is not allowed to mail Doctors Data test kits to any NJ, NY or RI address. I had to have them mail her kit to me in CA, and I flew to see her, get some of her hair to test and get her set up with glutathione to take on a daily basis to detoxify her and keep her safe. Because she was still on the independent side of the facility, we family by NJ law had to fill her vitamin and pill boxes with her vitamins and daily maintenance medication. Aides were allowed to open the lid for my mom but she had to take the meds/vits out and take her own daily vits and meds.

We purposely did NOT tell the aide service we were adding glutathione to her boxes because one particular nurses aide I pinpointed as the problem was still around my mom periodically from the service. (Note: the aide I complained about to the service finally fired her on December 23, 2019 after a few more incidents occurred – namely, my mother remembering the aide giving her a 'sleeping pill' from the aide's pocket, telling my mother it would help her 'sleep better'. NJ law forbids any aide giving a client medication of any sort from their person).

But the Doctors Data test clearly showed the high levels of zinc, copper, and uranium (!) in her body. (Note: there is a non-radioactive version of the uranium isotope that we believe our suspects used versus a radioactive version) Her hospital test from the Mayo Clinic in January 2019 was able to detect fair amounts of arsenic and cadmium in her system, so I knew those were issues as well.

Below are three Doctors Data test results on my mother taken February 22, 2019, five months later on July 22, 2019, and almost a year later on June 18, 2020 to show the effectiveness of glutathione as a detoxifier. NOTE: The aSquared brand of reduced glutathione was the ONLY detoxification element used to detoxify my mother. My mom has severe dementia and we did not want to complicate life for her by adding activated charcoal (which would easily be noticed in her pill box) or other detox methods. We had her taking 500mg in the morning (2 capsules at 250mg each) and 500mg in the evening. The capsules are smaller than most brands and easy for an older person to swallow, plus we liked that it looked like medication instead of a supplement so a particular nurses aide would not know it was a detox/immunity element.

You can see how amazing this non-liposomal version of reduced glutathione is in detoxifying the body! Liposomal is a more highly absorbable version of glutathione that most health practitioners recommend (I do as well) but in keeping things simple and be able to fit in my mother's vitamin/pill compartments easily, the aSquared brand still effectively detoxified my mother to get rid of her diarrhea, involuntary hand shaking, and nerve pain.

Also, no more fainting from lack of oxygen in the blood. ☺

> • • • <

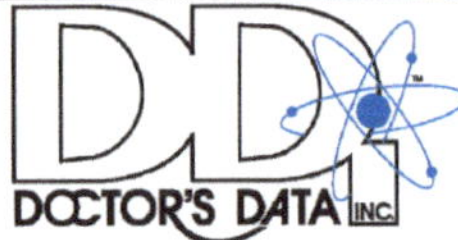

LAB #: H190225-2431-1
PATIENT: Agnes J. Padovan
ID: PADOVAN-A-00010
SEX: Female
AGE: 83

CLIENT #: 24237
DOCTOR: Anna Davis, MD
Direct Laboratory Services
4040 Florida St Ste 101
Mandeville, LA 70448 U.S.A.

Toxic Element Exposure Profile; Hair

TOXIC METALS		RESULT µg/g	REFERENCE INTERVAL	PERCENTILE 68th 95th
Arsenic	(As)	0.025	< 0.14	
Lead	(Pb)	1.3	< 3.0	
Mercury	(Hg)	0.49	< 3.0	
Cadmium	(Cd)	0.010	< 0.20	
Chromium	(Cr)	0.36	< 0.85	
Beryllium	(Be)	< 0.01	< 0.050	
Cobalt	(Co)	0.005	< 0.15	
Nickel	(Ni)	0.26	< 1.0	
Zinc	(Zn)	380	< 300	
Copper	(Cu)	110	< 70	
Thorium	(Th)	< 0.001	< 0.005	
Thallium	(Tl)	< 0.001	< 0.005	
Barium	(Ba)	0.08	< 8.0	
Cesium	(Cs)	< 0.002	< 0.010	
Manganese	(Mn)	0.18	< 1.5	
Selenium	(Se)	1.0	< 2.1	
Bismuth	(Bi)	0.057	< 5.0	
Vanadium	(V)	0.015	< 0.20	
Silver	(Ag)	0.16	< 1.6	
Antimony	(Sb)	0.018	< 0.12	
Palladium	(Pd)	0.004	< 0.015	
Aluminum	(Al)	7.3	< 19	
Platinum	(Pt)	< 0.003	< 0.010	
Tungsten	(W)	0.002	< 0.015	
Tin	(Sn)	0.06	< 1.0	
Uranium	(U)	3.4	< 0.20	
Gold	(Au)	0.027	< 0.50	
Tellurium	(Te)	< 0.05	< 0.050	
Germanium	(Ge)	0.034	< 0.045	
Titanium	(Ti)	0.30	< 2.0	
Gadolinium	(Gd)	< 0.001	< 0.008	

SPECIMEN DATA

Comments:

Date Collected: 02/22/2019
Date Received: 02/25/2019
Date Completed: 02/27/2019

Method: ICP-MS
<dl: less than detection limit
µg/g = ppm

Sample Type: **Head**
Sample Size: **0.163 g**
Hair Color:
Treatment:
Shampoo:

Metals are listed in descending priority order based upon data from the Agency for Toxic Substances and Disease Registry which considers not only the relative toxicity per gram metal, but also the frequency for occurrence of exposure.

This was the first forensic test through Doctors Data done on my mom to see where her levels were at and as proof of poisoning by showing how high these elements were in her. Note that the full amount of arsenic, cadmium didn't show and no thallium showed through at all. Note how high the uranium level is! 3.4 !

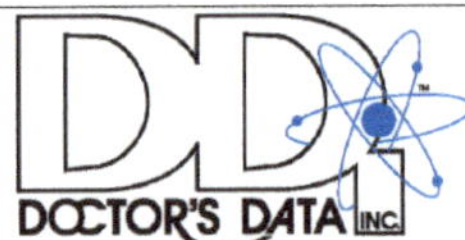

LAB #: H190725-2454-1
PATIENT: Agnes J. Padovan
ID: PADOVAN-A-00010
SEX: Female
DOB: 10/23/1935   **AGE:** 83

CLIENT #: 24237
DOCTOR: Anna Davis, MD
Direct Laboratory Services
4040 Florida St Ste 101
Mandeville, LA 70448 U.S.A.

Toxic Element Exposure Profile; Hair

TOXIC METALS		RESULT µg/g	REFERENCE INTERVAL	PERCENTILE 68th / 95th
Arsenic	(As)	0.048	< 0.14	
Lead	(Pb)	1.0	< 3.0	
Mercury	(Hg)	0.66	< 3.0	
Cadmium	(Cd)	0.036	< 0.20	
Chromium	(Cr)	0.44	< 0.85	
Beryllium	(Be)	< 0.01	< 0.050	
Cobalt	(Co)	0.002	< 0.15	
Nickel	(Ni)	0.13	< 1.0	
Zinc	(Zn)	150	< 300	
Copper	(Cu)	32	< 70	
Thorium	(Th)	< 0.001	< 0.005	
Thallium	(Tl)	< 0.001	< 0.005	
Barium	(Ba)	0.07	< 8.0	
Cesium	(Cs)	< 0.002	< 0.010	
Manganese	(Mn)	0.10	< 1.5	
Selenium	(Se)	0.90	< 2.1	
Bismuth	(Bi)	0.003	< 5.0	
Vanadium	(V)	0.042	< 0.20	
Silver	(Ag)	0.47	< 1.6	
Antimony	(Sb)	0.021	< 0.12	
Palladium	(Pd)	< 0.004	< 0.015	
Aluminum	(Al)	6.0	< 19	
Platinum	(Pt)	< 0.003	< 0.010	
Tungsten	(W)	0.001	< 0.015	
Tin	(Sn)	0.06	< 1.0	
Uranium	(U)	0.40	< 0.20	
Gold	(Au)	0.059	< 0.50	
Tellurium	(Te)	< 0.05	< 0.050	
Germanium	(Ge)	0.033	< 0.045	
Titanium	(Ti)	0.38	< 2.0	
Gadolinium	(Gd)	< 0.001	< 0.008	

SPECIMEN DATA

Comments:

Date Collected: 07/22/2019
Date Received: 07/25/2019
Date Reported: 07/31/2019

Method: ICP-MS
<dl: less than detection limit
µg/g = ppm

Sample Type: **Head**
Sample Size: **0.197 g**
Hair Color:
Treatment:
Shampoo:

Metals are listed in descending priority order based upon data from the Agency for Toxic Substances and Disease Registry which considers not only the relative toxicity per gram metal, but also the frequency for occurrence of exposure.

Exactly 5 months later. Note where her levels are in only 5 months, using the aSquared brand of reduced glutathione. Uranium now 0.4.

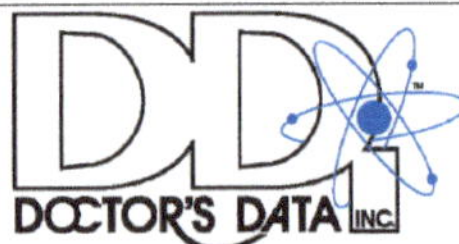

LAB #: H200629-2284-1
PATIENT: Agnes J. Padovan
ID: PADOVAN-A-00010
SEX: Female
DOB: 10/23/1935   **AGE:** 84

CLIENT #: 24237
DOCTOR: Aravinthan Suppiah, MD
Direct Laboratory Services
4040 Florida St Ste 101
Mandeville, LA 70448 U.S.A.

Toxic Element Exposure Profile; Hair

TOXIC METALS		RESULT μg/g	REFERENCE INTERVAL	PERCENTILE 68th	95th
Arsenic	(As)	0.072	< 0.14		
Lead	(Pb)	0.10	< 3.0		
Mercury	(Hg)	0.40	< 3.0		
Cadmium	(Cd)	0.025	< 0.20		
Chromium	(Cr)	0.51	< 0.85		
Beryllium	(Be)	< 0.01	< 0.050		
Cobalt	(Co)	0.002	< 0.15		
Nickel	(Ni)	0.06	< 1.0		
Zinc	(Zn)	160	< 300		
Copper	(Cu)	13	< 70		
Thorium	(Th)	< 0.001	< 0.005		
Thallium	(Tl)	< 0.001	< 0.005		
Barium	(Ba)	< 0.04	< 8.0		
Cesium	(Cs)	< 0.002	< 0.010		
Manganese	(Mn)	0.07	< 1.5		
Selenium	(Se)	0.80	< 2.1		
Bismuth	(Bi)	< 0.002	< 5.0		
Vanadium	(V)	0.077	< 0.20		
Silver	(Ag)	0.05	< 1.6		
Antimony	(Sb)	< 0.01	< 0.12		
Palladium	(Pd)	< 0.004	< 0.015		
Aluminum	(Al)	1.6	< 19		
Platinum	(Pt)	< 0.003	< 0.010		
Tungsten	(W)	0.001	< 0.015		
Tin	(Sn)	0.20	< 1.0		
Uranium	(U)	0.18	< 0.20		
Gold	(Au)	0.027	< 0.50		
Tellurium	(Te)	< 0.05	< 0.050		
Germanium	(Ge)	0.035	< 0.045		
Titanium	(Ti)	0.25	< 2.0		
Gadolinium	(Gd)	< 0.001	< 0.008		

SPECIMEN DATA

Comments:

Date Collected: 06/18/2020
Date Received: 06/29/2020
Date Reported: 07/02/2020

Method: ICP-MS
<dl: less than detection limit
μg/g = ppm

Sample Type: Head
Sample Size: 0.201 g
Hair Color:
Treatment:
Shampoo: Generic

Metals are listed in descending priority order based upon data from the Agency for Toxic Substances and Disease Registry which considers not only the relative toxicity per gram metal, but also the frequency for occurrence of exposure.

0001643   1731767

Almost a year later. By this time, our mother was down to 500mg a day of aSquared brand reduced glutathione. However, I noted her arsenic level was going up, which was a concern as the fired nurses aide was still in the building, working for another aide service, even with reassurance the aide wasn't supposed to go near my mother. We finally moved my mother out of the facility (no video cameras monitor residents) and did not tell the facility where we were moving her to for her safety.

Chapter 3:
The Protection of Glutathione on Active Covid-19

So how well does glutathione work on an active Covid-19 case? In the case of my mother, she was moved out of the family owned but very large, loosely monitored assisted living facility in NJ and moved to a much smaller, privately owned facility in another state close to some relatives. This was in October 2020 when Covid-19 was still an issue in many areas but moving was not a problem with proper arrangements. Even though stressful, I was able to fly her safely to her new home and make sure she was settled in comfortably.

Now I kept my mom on the aSquared brand at 500mg a day after those initial 5 months. Each capsule is only 250mg, so one in the morning and one in the evening. She was now completely in assisted living, so by law, only nurses with my mom's supplements and medication locked in the nurses' office were allowed to give her medication and her vitamin supplements.

Over Thanksgiving weekend in November 2020, all states were supposed to limit gatherings to keep the passing of virus germs to a minimum. My mom only went out of the building to see two relatives for dinner at their home and come straight back to the building, using full precautions – masks, waiting outside the building to pick her up, etc.

I was called the next day and asked how many people my mom saw for Thanksgiving. I said two. I made it clear they only went straight to their home, not to a restaurant, and brought her straight back. However, someone got confused with a staff member who actually went to a large gathering, and I was called again 2 days later, saying they were isolating my mother in her apartment because they were told she went to a large event. I said no, my mom saw only 2 people and didn't even go to a restaurant. There then was a panic in that they had isolated the wrong person, but I guess at that point, it was too late.

Residents started showing symptoms of flu or Covid-19 within a few days. The facility dining hall and all activities were closed to reduce transmission. However, the call came in mid-December 2020, to say my mother had now tested positive for Covid-19. By this time, all of the residents in the whole building (approximately 50) had been isolated in each of their apartments to restrict transmission.

To give you more of an idea how amazing glutathione is in protecting the body from having Covid-19 be fatal in an elderly person, my mother had had double bypass heart surgery with not one but two valve replacements 5 years prior to December 2020. She had turned 84 in October 2020, and considering her age and her prior heart surgery, you would think she would have suffered badly with Covid, maybe even have had to be hospitalized. In fact, she had been briefly hospitalized in late October 2020 when she received a Flu shot and had a horrible reaction – chills, then sweating, and low blood pressure. I found out the nurses were only giving her 250mg a day of her glutathione and I insisted they get it back to 500mg a day when she returned from the hospital. A call to her doctor also made that happen.

My mother barely cracked a fever on her 2nd day with Covid-19 (99 degrees, they said) and her only complaint was for fatigue which at her age was normal in general, but not surprising because she did have Covid. After that, normal temperature, oxygen levels normal and no other problems. Just a lot of rest – which she had to do because she wasn't allowed out of her apartment to even walk the hallways for at least 2 weeks.

In total, 39 of the 50 or so residents came down with Covid and 10 staff members also tested positive and when positive, had to isolate at home till they tested negative. Four (4) residents died, including the resident who was first to test positive.

Compared to many of the other residents who had severe symptoms, Covid was like a mild cold for my mom. But she was the only person in the building (and still is) who takes glutathione, and happens to have been on glutathione since February 2019 and yes, positively, absolutely, still takes it daily. (Hope to get more staffers and residents there in using glutathione for immunity boosting and for detoxifying).

I honestly don't know a better example of showing the detoxification and viral protection of glutathione than my own mom.

> • • • <

Chapter 4:
Protection from Covid-19 shots with Glutathione

Now you are going to say 'Ok, we can see with the studies and your example how glutathione protects the body from Covid and other viruses and illnesses in general, but what has that got to do with the Covid shots?'

Again, **everything**. Back toward the end of 2020, when Moderna, Johnson & Johnson, AstraZeneca and Pfizer were announcing they were getting ready to roll out the Emergency Authorization Use (EAU) of the Covid-19 'vaccines' worldwide, I had a touch base call with Dr. Staninger.

One of the first things she said was 'don't get the Covid shot!' I told her I absolutely had no plans to get any shots, especially because my body was now extremely sensitive to even a slight amount of toxicity, and with the mRNA and other high tech in the shots, I knew intuitively it wouldn't be good for me. Besides the fact that I took daily glutathione and knew I had viral protection. And also because Dr. S is in the know of everything that goes on and she intuitively felt the shots would be bad news – which unfortunately, turned out to be right.

Now towards the end of December 2020 and into the first week of January 2021, the facility my mom lived at received their free Covid shots from their state to distribute to their residents. I was called by the medical director since I am my mom's Power of Attorney to ask if I wanted my mom to get the first of 2 Covid shots.

'Absolutely, positively NOT', I told him. I explained she had had a horrible reaction to the Flu shot in late October 2020 and even had to go to the hospital for a couple of days to regulate her blood pressure.

AND she had just recovered from Covid and was on daily glutathione, a proven viral protectant, so at this time, I felt getting any type of shot was too risky.

So at that time, she didn't get any Covid-19 shots of any kind.

Fast forward to June 2021. My siblings are very much products of believing anything mainstream media says to them. The new Delta variant was making the rounds around the world, and my siblings were very frightened from all the news they were listening to. They felt our mom needed extra protection and they wanted her to get the shots.

I explained she already went through Covid in December 2020 and was on glutathione for protection. They insisted they wanted her to get the shots because Delta appeared even more deadly (they all got the shots – nothing I could say or do to stop them on that).

Because it's 3 of them and 1 of me, and I do believe in a democracy, I said ok, but that it was a huge risk. There had been news now that people had shown adverse reactions to one or more Covid shots which matched the same symptoms I, my mom and others had when we had heavy metal poisoning. I felt there definitely was something going on. There was a risk our mom could react badly.

Again, outvoted so I said ok, and now there were no free shots available at the facility, so relatives took our mom in late June 2021 to get her first Moderna shot at a local Walgreens pharmacy. Remember, she is still taking 500mg daily of glutathione (I periodically checked the facility to make sure that was the case) of the aSquared reduced glutathione. I asked the facility to watch her like a hawk to see if she was going to show any adverse reaction and if so, I would ask to bump up her glutathione. Our mom showed no reaction – no fever, no diarrhea, no breathing issues.

She then had the 2nd Moderna shot in November 2021. Again, I asked the facility to watch her carefully for any bad reactions. She showed no reactions to getting the shot.

I credit the glutathione in keeping her body in a detoxified state, so that if there were any toxins in those particular shots, the glutathione levels in her body most likely kept flowing the toxins out of her, keeping them from her heart and other vital organs.

The other added benefit with the long-term use of glutathione for my mom is it restored her ability to be more independent again. When she first arrived at the facility in early October 2020, the nurse rated her care at Level 4. A few months later, I received a call and was told they were reducing my mom's care level to Level 3.

By December 2021, I received a call from the facility's manager, saying my mom's level of care had now gone down to Level 2 ! Meaning she was fully capable of showering and dressing herself without any assistance from a staffer! Incredible!

The only thing I will say that made me think there may have been some residual toxicity from the shots was around February 2022, our mom had come downstairs to breakfast with one side of her face bruised. She was asked what happened, and she said she fell against the shower wall, getting out of the shower.

Unfortunately, since she was alone, no one can say whether her old slippers slipped on the bathroom rug as she got out, or did she actually faint and hit the wall. With her dementia, she is unsure of what exactly happened.

So as a precaution, I changed her glutathione brand to Jarrows because their brand has 500mg per capsule and asked the nurse to bump up our mom's glutathione intake to 500mg twice a day. For now, she is still taking 1000mg a day for detoxification and immune support.

Plus she got new slippers and a better, non-slip bathroom rug ☺ .

> • • • <

Bad Shot? ASAP: Detox!   p 36

Chapter 5:
Forensic proof of toxins in the Covid shots

So now here we are towards the tail end of 2022. There has been tremendous amounts of news on how damaging the Covid shots have been. Numerous doctors speaking out about the dangers of the shots, many getting fired or losing their positions at hospitals for doing so. Numerous Covid shot injured groups springing up all over the world. Almost every law firm out there, creating lawsuits, looking to get their clients compensation for their injuries.

I knew after I safely got out of California that I needed to go public with this information – what I and my family went through in connection to the similarities to adverse reactions to the Covid shots, and tell people to get properly forensically tested, but most important even before testing was to start detoxifying the toxicity in the body.

Now I have been trying since 2017 to get interviewed on news stations as to what we were going through with being poisoned and how our suspects were using nano tech to hide the metal toxins from view in regular doctor and hospital tests, and the concern they were going to do this on a grander scale and make lots of money through doctors and pharmacies they were connected with, to keep people suffering and paying for treatment that would make symptoms worse (heavy metals will interfere with any harsh gastro intestinal or any very heavy medication taken). Plus the problems I was having getting the FBI to cooperate with helping our police and allow the use of their forensic labs that FBI told me in 2017, any police could use if they asked. (You know with recent news what's going on with the FBI).

Being a nobody in a sense, no one would even call me or email me back on all the forensics and proof I showed that this was a serious issue. So I started making videos and posting them on YouTube to educate the public on heavy metal toxicity, showing examples of our forensic tests, with before and after results detoxifying with glutathione. The rub came when YouTube specifically would not allow any videos that so much as hinted that the Covid shots were possibly a problem, let alone completely a problem.

Where can you go to post without censorship? Rumble.com to name one of a few media sites still freely allowing those to post whatever they wish. So I went there and started a channel:

https://rumble.com/c/ThePaladina

The first video on Rumble.com that went up was February 8, 2022 with this subject header: **Covid shots: side effects = heavy metal symptoms. Important to detox now to recover**

Imagine seeing that on YouTube! Actually it was pulled off YouTube for being 'misinformation' and I received my first warning. Even just saying that side effects matched heavy metal symptoms (true statement) wasn't allowed.

I then went on to creating several important videos in February 2022, showing full panel forensic tests, before and after detox of allergy tests, a client's toxicity clinic test showing the amount of liver impairment, low hormone count and even parasite infections in her body but how the test could not show the toxins because the test had no forensic modalities to bypass the nano. Comparing a full panel toxicity test revealing everything against hospital tests revealing nothing.

Though I feel one of the most important videos I put together was

COVID-19 shot adverse effects - You can fully heal!

Detoxify even nano tech Video link:

https://rumble.com/vuvcju-covid-19-long-haul-and-shot-adverse-effects-you-can-fully-heal.html

Imagine being told by your doctor that you will 'always' have this problem of ulcerated colitis or myocarditis or Crohn's Disease or any number of illnesses – all because your doctor will not test you for toxicity and get you to detoxify to recover. Making $$ keeping you sick.

But even more important: even if your doctor tested you for metal or chemical toxins, _nothing will show on the doctor's tests because the nano tech will hide it from view_. It has to be a full forensic, comprehensive heavy metals and chemicals and unknown toxins test, if you really want to see the toxins in your body.

What I was relaying to people in the video is you can fully heal if you removed the toxins and nano tech from the body just like I did and glutathione was not only the answer to remove metals, chemicals and nanobots safely from the body, but also was a viral protector against Covid-19. I included study links, test website, doctor protocols and supplement recommendations in all video descriptions to help people out.

But the biggest information now that I brought forward on September 11, 2022, the anniversary of 9/11 was

Toxic Substances Found in COVID Vaccines "Without Exception" - new German study

https://rumble.com/v1jodlh-toxic-substances-found-in-covid-vaccines-without-exception-new-german-study.html

Here was the kicker. New forensic testing done by The Working Group for COVID Vaccine Analysis in Germany found heavy metal elements in Moderna, Pfizer and AstraZeneca vaccine vials. "Anomalous" objects were found in the Johnson & Johnson's Janssen vector vaccine but not found in all the J & J samples.

Full article at this link: https://www.momsacrossamerica.com/toxic_substances_found_in_covid_vaccines

"The following metallic elements were found in the vaccines:

- **Alkali metals: cesium (Cs), potassium (K)**

- **Alkaline earth metals: calcium (Ca), barium (Ba)**

- **Transition metals: cobalt (Co), iron (Fe), chromium (Cr), titanium (Ti)**

- **Rare earth metals: cerium (Ce), gadolinium (Gd)**

- **Mining group/metal: aluminum (Al)**

- **Carbon group: silicon (Si) (partly support material/ slide)**

- **Oxygen group: sulfur (S)**

Gastrointestinal and kidney dysfunction, nervous system disorders, skin lesions, vascular damage, immune system dysfunction, congenital disabilities, and cancer are the complications of heavy metals' toxic effects.

Bioaccumulation of these heavy metals leads to diverse toxic effects on various body tissues and organs. Heavy metals disrupt cellular events, including growth, proliferation, differentiation, damage-repairing processes, and apoptosis. A comparison of the mechanisms of action reveals similar pathways for these metals to induce toxicity, including ROS generation, weakening of the antioxidant defense, enzyme inactivation, and oxidative stress."

*Mom's Across America article insert Aug 2022

How bad is this? It's bad, believe me. If people don't detoxify their bodies from the toxins, nano tech, anomalous objects and spike proteins, worsening conditions can lead to cancer and death. What also was worth noting was seeing 5 of the metal elements listed were what our suspects used on us besides the addition of other metals in varying combinations.

So here was proof that I was correct. Adverse reactions were matching heavy metal symptoms for a reason: heavy metals were actually present.

Now I don't care that I'm correct. I care that it is even more urgent now to get people tested and detoxified before more deaths and more suffering continues.

> • • • <

Bad Shot? ASAP: Detox!   p 42

Chapter 6:

Nano technology, forensic testing and detoxifying

'Ok, Christine – so what do I do if I had a Covid shot and I did go through some symptoms?' Detoxify. **I'm not kidding.** You just saw the listing of metal elements found in forensic testing. Feel free to read the entire article on MomsAcrossAmerica.com which includes photos. The photos alone will convince you of the importance of detoxifying. I provide that great video with supplement recommendations on detoxifying on Rumble.com (see link again in Chapter 5) and you can get more detox methods and information at https://heavymetalpoisoncenter.com

Anyone who had even one Covid shot, whether they had adverse reactions or not, even just minor fatigue, needs to detoxify their bodies. Why? Because every single shot has nanobots in them and a nanobot can be programmed to create a delayed or even slow release. So some people have immediate reactions, and we have seen others with delayed reactions. The fainting is a great example of that.

We actually saw this in action when my former lover was poisoned after going to a family event the suspect hosted at their home in March 2018. I and a cousin of his, with her own personal experience with this suspect, begged him not to go. He went – naively saying 'oh, she knows now she's being investigated. (Side note: Corrupt detective in the new town she moved to told her I was investigating her – that put a big monkey wrench in all our cases and made me more of a target). So she won't hurt me in front of people.'

Really? Just so you know, if a sociopath or psychopath has it out for you, and they are a skilled poisoner with substances that are odorless, colorless and tasteless, they will charmingly offer you food or drink with a smile, even an empty tainted glass or plate, even with other people around and inside themselves, they are gleeful that you are such a trusting smuck to let them do this to you.

Within 3 days from that event, he was in the hospital. White cell count through the roof, red cell count through the floor, thrombosis in the legs and clots in the lungs. Of course, the raging, bloody diarrhea, nausea, stomach pain. Many of you have gone through this.

Now at that time in March 2018, I didn't know nano tech was being used to keep the elements from being seen in doctor tests. I thought because we may have waited too long in between poisoning events for my loved one and the urine tests we did were negative because the elements were now out of the urinary tract and deeper inside tissue, organs and hair. So I had then done expensive forensic tests on hair to show the proof that I was intuitively correct. (You try to tell someone they should test for toxins and sometimes you get 'nah, can't be that.' Many people do not want to believe this could happen to them and instead of facing reality, then go into denial. You know the story - you can lead a horse to water but …

I thought – ok, at least because the poisoning just occurred, it will show in urine and blood tests at the hospital to prove this person was poisoned (note: toxins only stay in blood for a week, then pass on through the urinary tract for between 6 to 8 weeks, after that the toxins will continue to settle in tissues and organs, but can be seen through forensic hair testing).

Were the toxins seen on the hospital tests? **NO.** I showed our 2017 forensic tests and insisted on at least arsenic and thallium tests for blood, since the event occurred only 3 days prior and those were 2 main elements always used by our suspects. Should still see the elements in the blood, right? Not with nanobots hiding it. (Note: our suspects as you saw with some of our tests used many different metals in varying degrees on all of us. Hospitals do not do full panel testing so you have to ask for each element you want tested. Another reason to make full panel forensic metal and chemical testing a standard in the medical industry)

I thought 'Great! Now we'll also have hospital proof because this poisoning happened only a couple of days ago'. Yet NO thallium showed at all and only 7 ug/L of arsenic showed through!

I called Dr. Staninger and asked was there something that could mask the metals from being seen on these hospital tests. She said yes, **nanobots** could do that and keep the metals or any toxin from being seen on standard LabCorp, Quest Diagnostics or even Mayo Clinic tests as I did later for my mother when she was hospitalized for mysterious and suspicious fainting at her assisted living place in NJ.

The other interesting factor was when a urine test was done 10 days later on arsenic and thallium. Now the arsenic level showed through at 21 ug/L. But thallium of course showed nothing. While in the hospital, away from the suspects.

I asked Dr. Staninger then – could the nanobots do a slow release of the toxins in the body, so people will not know they were poisoned by a certain person or medication because it happened so far in the past?

She said **YES**, absolutely. Nano technology can be programmed to do anything. She had seen similar occurrences in other poisoning cases. And yes, the other possibility is someone was paid to add more to him, but the police had been called so they and I were watching him very carefully.

Doesn't mean it's not possible but the more likely reason is a slow release of toxins gotten from the family event.

After getting out of the hospital, he finally agreed to do serious detoxification and finally stay away from this particular in-law.

In a nutshell, any testing methods used by doctors or hospitals do not have forensic modalities to bypass nano technology and give a full, complete picture of all metals and chemicals in the body. Imagine how frustrating it is, trying to convince doctors that your loved one is full of toxicity by showing prior forensic proof, but having those doctors not believe you because **their current** tests show nothing.

The other big reason to detoxify is what I just mentioned. Possible slow release of toxins by nano technology, programmed to release or activate at different times.

> • • • <

Chapter 7:
An Affordable Forensic Lab Resource for Tests

So, you ask - what's the best way to get tested without going broke, paying possibly thousands of dollars per test like you did, if my insurance doesn't cover toxicology tests?

I researched a more affordable solution to this problem as I also wanted a future resource that would not cost thousands per test. I also wanted tests for people that didn't just have one forensic modality or could not be mailed to particular states or countries. The public needed full panel, full modality forensic testing that was available anywhere and everywhere.

The answer currently is Directlabs. They are a U.S. nationwide company with a digital, online presence and have the ability to mail test kits to 47 states (exception for now being NJ, NY and RI because of some laws not allowing health kits from outside the state but we offer you a way to get the test through our company in FL as a mailing source). Their Hair Toxic Element Exposure-Doctor's Data Kit for Heavy Metals (offered for urine and hair) is a full forensic ICP-MS test (Inductively Coupled Plasma Spectroscopy with Mass Spectrometry). Their Environmental Pollutants Profile (EPP) (Dried Urine)-US BioTek Kit utilizes Gas Chromatography and Mass Spectrometry in uncovering chemical-based toxins in the body. Both methods bypass any nano tech to reveal everything.

This is very important in bypassing any nano tech and revealing everything that is inside of you. Directlabs can offer you a testing slip to take to any Quest Diagnostics lab near you to take your sample for you to mail back to Directlabs, or you can be mailed a test kit to do it yourself. All tests include Chain of Custody and are admissible in court, if needed for criminal or civil cases. (Note: there are many groups such as Freedom Flyers suing employers for forcing employees to get Covid shots because they are now unable to do their jobs. You need to prove you have toxicity from one or more Covid shots in you, not just show tests showing injury. Also, please detoxify to recover).

Another plus: Directlabs can mail a test kit **anywhere in the world**. That is a wonderful thing since billions of people have gotten one or more Covid shots who may want to prove to themselves or a doctor that they have toxins in their body, and they need to detoxify. Or want proof for a lawsuit. There is also toxicity in general happening environmentally and accidentally besides intentionally - these tests can be taken for any reason, not just for adverse reactions to a shot.

These test kits are as affordable as possible, in case you don't have insurance, or your insurance doesn't cover this type of testing. (Another thing I'm trying to change – having all insurance cover toxicology testing and treatment). Directlabs can provide insurance CPT codes and a CPT receipt if you do have insurance and wish to submit for possible reimbursement.

The forensic toxicity tests currently range between $124.00 and $169.00, depending on the type of test (metals or chemicals and if any discounts/coupons are available online). Outside the U.S., ask for pricing. A comprehensive test for chemicals, food additives, molds and more called ELISA/Act Basic is listed for $499.99. Lower priced tests are listed for food allergies (which toxicity causes allergic reactions to numerous food temporarily until you detoxify), hormone testing, vitamin D testing and other general health tests.

Another reason to use Directlabs – besides giving you a full report for your records, we're trying to collect the forensic proof that Covid shots are putting toxins in people (all information stays confidential) and have little to no benefit in stopping Covid-19 transmissions and illnesses. We want to stop mandates and distribution of shots as they have not proven to stop Covid-19 and have caused more harm than good to humanity. Besides, we have a natural solution with supplements such as glutathione and adequate levels of vitamin D offering protection against viruses.

You can contact Directlab from our special testing page here: https://www.directlabs.com/thepaladina - use code R-PALA for orders

Or call 1-800-908-0000 (U.S.) for assistance in ordering a full panel forensic toxicity test and reference code R-PALA. If testing for Covid shot toxicity, we recommend the Doctors Data Toxic Elements for metals test (if shots taken within 6 weeks of testing, urine is fine. After 6 weeks, hair is best for test purposes). If you wish to do only 1 test or can afford only 1 test, we recommend the metals (toxic elements) forensic test since metals have been found in forensic testing of Covid shot formulas. Hair, nails and even ashes can be tested of a deceased loved one (human or animal) to prove what killed them. Forensic testing is that sophisticated now. (Note below on specialty testing).

The other benefit we provide is a **FREE** report analysis and initial detox consult (a $325.00 value) when you share your results with us plus this helps us get more data on how many people have been harmed by CV shots and/or other medical shots. Just add Paladina International and our contact email - christine@thepaladina.com to your order form. (We are HIPAA certified and insured - all private info stays confidential)

Again, our special page link to our toxicologist recommended tests: https://www.directlabs.com/thepaladina or if ordering online, the listing of tests are here: https://store.directlabs.com/rs/Pala

Or call the special number 1-800-908-0000 and use code R-PALA and ask for assistance in placing an order. (Please add our name Paladina Int'l and email christine@thepaladina.com to your HIPAA order form or ask Directlabs to do this, so you can share your results with us- again, we provide FREE analysis consults; HIPAA certified staff)

NOTE: Directlabs cannot do specialty testing for animal fur or finger/ toe nails. This can be done through The Carlson Company at

https://thecarlsoncompany.net/ - we have done such testing to prove poisoning in a water tank intentionally tainted; poisoning of a beloved pet, ourselves and more for police cases. When you call them, mention Christine Padovan and receive special reduced pricing. These are higher in price (normally 1750, but as low as 1195 mentioning my name) and do not provide insurance codes, but results are phenomenal. Also, admissible in court.

I provided an example of my mom's toxicity tests from Directlabs in this video.

https://rumble.com/v2lcnaq-directlabs-forensic-toxicity-tests-at-even-lower-pricing-lets-stoptheshots.html

Clients have provided their tests. Check back frequently to

https://rumble.com/c/ThePaladina for future videos on people's tests.

In the near future, as I gain sponsors for my media show and partnerships in taking my company worldwide in educating the public, and the medical industry in all countries on the importance of detoxifying any type of toxicity from the body to stay healthy, I plan to put money into providing free forensic testing to those who completely cannot afford a test, even as we get pricing lower over time.

I fully believe all of what I went through was to learn how heavy metal toxins, especially those hidden by nano tech, can fool doctors into believing your symptoms and illnesses are naturally caused, and the importance of forensic testing to see if toxins are the root cause of the illness. FYI: Toxicity, whether mental, emotional or physical, is the root cause to almost any disease or illness.

But even more important is teaching people to be their own best advocate when it comes to their health, as most allopathic doctors are happy to just treat symptoms with medication and harsh treatment and never, ever digging deeper to uncover exactly why you are ill. Even many of the doctors you see being interviewed on television or radio, who are brave enough to say how bad the Covid shots are – many of them are happy to show the public the tests showing the damage and injury to someone's body, but many will not test the person or even if they do, test the person forensically to reveal **the reason behind** the sustained damage or injury from one or more Covid shots.

If your doctor is not having you get forensically tested to see if any toxins can be the underlying cause of your ulcerated colitis, your blood clots, your thrombosis, and even other severe injury or disease, how good is that doctor in healing you? Especially if the answer is to detoxify the toxins to restore your health?

I see in the next few years more people taking control of their health and finding their own answers that have always been the answer to illnesses and diseases: from nature and health practitioners who want their clients to be healthy and happy. I see pharmaceutical companies in the future going back to using naturopathic remedies in providing cures to illness and disease. Treating root cause, and not just the symptom. I see more people using mental, emotional and spiritual healing as well for whole body health. See my website https://thepaladina.com on those modalities.

I truly see the world becoming a better place – yes, I see world peace in the future – as we come together to help each other out, spread kindness and love, and help get through all the events currently going on in the world.

We will get through this, believe me. I love you all! Contact my company if you need further assistance and support.

> • • • <

Recent Questions from the Public and Answers:

Question: I heard the mRNA technology in the shots changes our DNA. So even if I detoxify, doesn't my DNA stay changed?

Answer: Good news! NO, it does not. Dr. Staninger confirmed that mRNA could affect a small portion of our DNA when it is programmed to do what it does. However, when the chemical used by mRNA (and any spike proteins) is removed from the DNA through detoxification (glutathione being the key element to pull it out), the DNA repairs itself and is restored. So those who received one or more shots and experienced mood swings, confusion, depression, sudden violent outbursts, suicidal thoughts and other behavioral changes besides other possible symptoms will go away when the person detoxifies. We have seen this from first hand accounts in our families.

Question: Can graphene oxide, nanobots, heavy metals and these anomalous objects really be removed safely from the body?

Answer: YES! Glutathione is an element in every cell of our bodies. It pulls out metals, chemicals, plastics, pollutants, stress, even alcohol from our bodies:

https://www.ncbi.nlm.nih.gov/pmc/articles/PMC4684116/

We were poisoned with heavy metals hidden from view by nano tech. We got it all out, even the nano (again, nano is either some form of polymer plastic and/or metal).

Question: What about using zeolite for detoxifying?

Answer: Zeolite is **never** recommended, despite the advertising you see on it. Zeolite is made of sodium aluminosilicate powders. It is not water-soluble like Vitamin C and Glutathione, and the other problem is there are too many unsafe, poor quality zeolite products out there. Trying to decide how much to take without causing detox issues of moving metals and other toxins too quickly could shock the body - possibly causing death from the shock.

Dr. Staninger said this about zeolite and why she does not use it or recommend it: "Some zeolites are used in nano. I do not use it because it has changed many formulas.

We also do not recommend hydro shots (hydrogen shots) or colloidal silver for detoxifying. However, Infrared sauna therapy and hyperbaric oxygen sessions are great additions to your detox program if you can afford them.

Question: Can you recommend some brands that have worked for you and are still quality and affordable?

Answer: Below you will find links to some of our preferred supplements that we and our clients have used with great success. Our company does not sell any products. This list is a free resource we have created in the hope it will make your life a little easier. To defray the costs associated with hosting these links, our company may earn a small commission for the sale of these products. Your purchase also helps support our work in providing you information about health and holistic wellness.

All non GMO and 3rd party verified. For full listing of supplements: https://thepaladina.com/health-wellness-orders.html

If money is tight and you want more product in your purchase but still of quality, we successfully used aSquared Nutrition's brand to continue detoxing ourselves and my mom when money became tight from mounting med and treatment bills. Each capsule is 250mg and in a smaller, easier to swallow form, so you customize how much you take. aSquared Nutrition also provides discount codes for bulk purchases (scroll through the photos on the left side of their page for the codes): https://amzn.to/3rAQ5F1

———————

Question: Isn't liposomal glutathione the best type to take?

Answer: Yes, in a sense. It is more highly absorbed in the body. We started out using the more expensive Core Med Science brand because that is what the local homeopathic doctor recommended, but being in liquid form, the taste is hard to tolerate for some people and it is expensive and since we had to do this long term, I researched regular supplement form brands of glutathione that were quality but more affordable. We still detoxified fine using a standard capsule form of reduced glutathione (aSquared Nutrition and Nusapure).

———————

Question: Isn't 'reduced' glutathione less effective? Why is it sold as reduced glutathione?

Answer: This is a science term. Glutathione, in its oxidized state, no longer functions as an antioxidant. Only if it is reduced, meaning it contains needed electrons, can glutathione effectively function as an antioxidant. This also makes it active. So you will see glutathione supplements listed as 'Reduced Glutathione' or GSH or L-glutathione and that is the formula to get.

Question: Why not just take NAC (N-acetyl cysteine) to boost your Glutathione levels in your body?

Answer: Regarding taking NAC in what people believe to be a glutathione booster or creator, Dr. Jimmy Gutman is a long-time medical doctor and consultant on glutathione and he wrote in 2002, that 'NAC-induced glutathione levels reach a rapid peak and decline within hours' and that to maintain glutathione levels, NAC must be swallowed or injected several times a day - which is hard on the body. It is also considered a chemical drug, used primarily for Tylenol overdoses and can have more side effects.

We personally do not recommend NAC as protection against viruses since it is not a fully natural substance. We recommend foods high in glutathione (bay leaves as bay leaf water, avocado, cilantro, etc.) and a quality glutathione supplement. But use of NAC along with glutathione have been studied in assisting glutathione in being a more effective detoxifier in pulling certain toxins out of the body such as mercury, so short term use can be beneficial for detoxification - though our toxicologist never recommended its use, only glutathione.

But if you go to Dr. Horowitz's link provided in Chapter 2, you will see his protocol includes NAC and glutathione used together for viral protection and recovery. So if you feel you wish to do both, that is up to you.

Just know that NAC used by itself to create glutathione in your body is **not** a benefit when it comes to detoxification or viral protections for the reasons Dr. Gutman stated above. Again, we personally don't use it nor recommend it.

Note: NAC is used in emergencies to prevent overdoses such as from cocaine or heroin or Tylenol. So if you or someone you know uses harsh medication or illicit drugs, it is probably a good idea to have a bottle of NAC on hand.

Christine Padovan is a Renaissance woman – a blend of both science and spiritual gifts. Her discovery of a group of people slow poisoning her and others with heavy metal toxins hidden by nanotechnology has led to her creation of

https://heavymetalpoisoncenter.com

and

https://thepaladina.com

in educating the world on how toxicity creates artificial illnesses and early death in people, and changing the medical and law enforcement fields in thoroughly testing victims and clients with forensic style tests that uncover all hidden toxic elements in the body, so the individual can be properly treated through safe, natural detoxification methods.

Her company, Paladina International is building a worldwide education presence to teach all countries on the importance of uncovering the source of, protecting from and detoxifying toxicity. Call 1-888-307-6780 or email christine@thepaladina.com if interested in business partnerships, individual or group consults/training or seminar/webinar engagements.

The company also accepts donations in helping provide free testing, media coverage and for company security:

https://www.paypal.com/donate/?hosted_button_id=AM8A522DE2P2

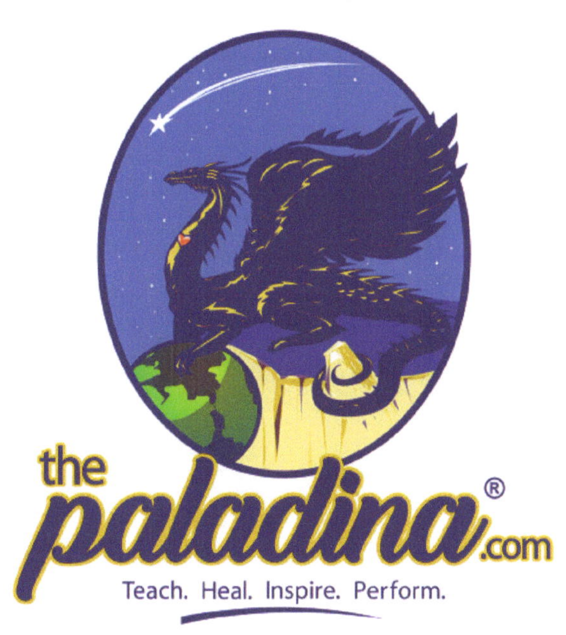
the
paladina®
.com
Teach. Heal. Inspire. Perform.